Copyright 20

MW01609019

This document is geared ....g ....
reliable information in regards to the topic and issue covered. The publication is sold on the idea that the publisher is not required to render an accounting, officially permitted, or otherwise, qualified services. If advice is necessary, legal or professional, a practiced individual in the profession should be ordered.

From a Declaration of Principles which was accepted and approved equally by a Committee of the American Bar Association and a Committee of Publishers and Associations.

1

Table of Contents

Introduction

I want to thank you and congratulate you on downloading this book. In this book you will learn delicious and healthy ways to prepare smoothies that are perfect for diabetics, however, everyone will enjoy it and its benefits.

The biggest concern that diabetics have is the sugar content in fruits. It's true that fruit contains glucose, and you should monitor your sugar and carbohydrate intake, however, you can enjoy fruits and greens.

In fact, green smoothies that you find in this book is proven to yield many benefits for people suffering from diabetes. Smoothies can boost weight loss, increase energy levels and improve your overall health, in turn, relieving diabetes condition. People have reported that drinking green smoothies allowed them to lose 20-50 pounds and some even managed to get off insulin.

In this book, you'll find lots of delicious and healthy smoothie recipes to choose from. Just drink one or two a day and you'll begin to see the results.

Of course, healthy nutrition, exercise and constant monitoring of your state are necessary, so don't treat smoothies as a magic pill that allows continuing eating all the food that got you into this condition. However, the smoothies you'll make here are an amazing and delicious way to improve your health, so enjoy!

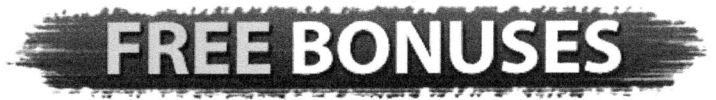

FREE BONUSES

Every copy of this book comes packed with 2 invaluable bonuses for diabetics and pre-diabetics:

BONUS #1: *Step-By-Step Blueprint* ***"6 Steps To Reverse Diabetes Naturally And Have A Perfect Health"*** *- FREE INSTANT DOWNLOAD*
BONUS #2: *Our exclusive newsletter subscription where we share tips, strategies and support to destroy diabetes once and for all - FREE INSTANT ACCESS*

Simply visit the special link below and enter your name & email address to get instant access.

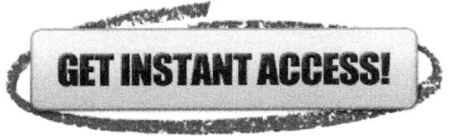

WWW.SOURCEOFHEALTHY.COM/6STEPS

Cherry-Blueberry Banana Smoothie

INGREDIENTS

- 1 1/2 cups frozen unsweetened pitted dark sweet or sour cherries
- 1 cup unsweetened vanilla-flavored almond milk
- 1 6 - ounce package Greek non-fat yogurt
- 1/2 cup fresh or frozen unsweetened blueberries
- 1 small banana, peeled

DIRECTIONS

1. In a blender combine cherries, milk, yogurt, blueberries, and banana. Cover and blend until smooth.
2. Pour into glasses to serve and enjoy!

Carrot-Mango Green Tea Smoothie

INGREDIENTS

- 3 cups water
- 1 cup sliced carrots or packaged peeled baby carrots
- 1 inch fresh ginger, thinly sliced
- 4 green tea bags
- 2 cups frozen mango chunks
- 1 teaspoon honey
- 1 tablespoon chia seeds (optional)

DIRECTIONS

1. In a small saucepan bring water to boiling. Add carrots; cover and cook for 10 to 15 minutes or until very tender, adding ginger slices for the last 2 minutes of cooking. Remove from the heat and add tea bags. Cover and steep for 4 minutes.
2. Remove tea bags, squeezing out all the tea. Remove ginger slices. Set pan on a hot pad in the refrigerator for 10 minutes.
3. Transfer carrot mixture to a blender. Add mango, honey, and chia (if using). Cover and blend until smooth.
4. Pour into glasses to serve and enjoy!

Mix-and-Match Banana Berry Smoothie

INGREDIENTS

- 1 medium banana, cut up
- 1 cup blueberries, raspberries, blackberries, or strawberries
- 1 cup frozen unsweetened peach slices
- 1/2 cup pomegranate, cherry, blueberry, or cranberry juice
- 1/2 cup low-fat plain or vanilla soymilk
- 1 cup ice cubes
- 1/4 cup low-fat granola
- 1/4 cup blueberries, raspberries, blackberries, or strawberries

DIRECTIONS

1. In a blender combine banana, 1 cup berries, peaches, fruit juice, and soymilk. Cover and blend until smooth. With the motor running, add ice cubes, one at a time, through the opening in the lid until combined and slushy.
2. Top each serving with granola and 1/4 cup berries. Enjoy!

Just Peachy Smoothie

INGREDIENTS

- 1 (6 ounces) package peach fat-free yogurt
- 1 cup fat-free milk
- 2 cups sliced fresh peaches, nectarines, and/or apricots
- 1 cup small ice cubes or crushed ice

DIRECTIONS

1. In a blender, combine yogurt, milk, and fruit. Cover and blend until smooth. Add ice; cover and blend until almost smooth.
2. Enjoy!

Chocolate-Banana Sipper

INGREDIENTS

- 2 cups fat-free milk
- 1 banana, sliced and frozen
- 3 tablespoons unsweetened cocoa powder
- 2 tablespoons honey
- 1 teaspoon vanilla

DIRECTIONS

1. In a blender, combine milk, banana, cocoa powder, honey, and vanilla. Cover and blend until smooth and frothy.
2. Enjoy!

Carrot Smoothie

INGREDIENTS

- 1 cup sliced carrots
- 1/2 teaspoon finely shredded orange peel
- 1 cup orange juice
- 1 1/2 cups ice cubes
- Orange peel curls (optional)

DIRECTIONS

1. In a covered small saucepan, cook carrots in a small amount of boiling water about 15 minutes or until very tender. Drain well. Cool.
2. Place drained carrots in a blender. Add finely shredded orange peel and orange juice. Cover and blend until smooth. Add ice cubes; cover and blend until smooth.
3. Pour into glasses and enjoy!

Strawberry-Banana Smoothie

INGREDIENTS

- 4 cups sliced fresh strawberries
- 1 medium banana, sliced
- 1 6 - ounce carton vanilla low-fat yogurt
- 1 cup ice cubes

DIRECTIONS

1. In a blender, combine strawberries, banana, and yogurt; cover and blend until smooth. With blender running, add ice cubes, one at a time, through a hole in the lid; blend until smooth.
2. Enjoy!

Sunrise Smoothie

INGREDIENTS

- 1 1/2 cups seeded, cut-up watermelon
- 1 cup cut-up cantaloupe
- 1/2 cup plain low-fat yogurt
- 1/4 cup orange juice

DIRECTIONS

1. Place the 1 1/2 cups watermelon in a blender. Cover and blend until smooth. Divide watermelon puree between two 12-ounce glasses; set aside. Rinse out the blender.
2. In a blender, combine the 1 cup cantaloupe, the yogurt, and orange juice. Cover and blend until smooth.
3. Slowly pour into glasses on top of watermelon puree.
4. Enjoy!

Peachy Apricot Slush

INGREDIENTS

- 1 5 1/2 - ounce can apricot nectar, chilled
- 2 medium peaches, peeled, pitted, and sliced
- 1 1/2 cups crushed ice
- 1 tablespoon lemon juice or lime juice
- 1 1/2 cups carbonated water, chilled

DIRECTIONS

1. In a blender, combine apricot nectar, peaches, crushed ice, and lemon or lime juice. Cover and blend until smooth.
2. Spoon fruit mixture into tall, chilled glasses; top with carbonated water.
3. Enjoy!

Harvest Time Sweet Potato Smoothie

INGREDIENTS

- 1/2 cup unsweetened almond milk
- 1/2 banana, frozen if you want a chilled smoothie
- 1/2 cup of sweet potato, cooked and peeled
- 1 tablespoon of peanut butter or almond butter
- 1/4 teaspoon cinnamon to taste

DIRECTIONS

1. Combine all ingredients in a blender and puree until smooth and thick.
2. Enjoy!

Green Smoothie

INGREDIENTS

- 1/2 cup unsweetened almond milk
- 1 small orange, peeled but with much of the pith left
- 1 cup spinach
- 1/2 cup frozen berries (blueberries, strawberries, raspberries)
- 1/2 cup Greek yogurt

DIRECTIONS

1. Combine all ingredients in a blender and puree until smooth and thick.
2. Enjoy!

Orange Green Smoothie

INGREDIENTS

- 1 small orange, peeled
- 2 big handfuls of spinach
- 1 large kale
- 1/2 cup frozen mixed berries
- 1 serving vegan protein powder
- 1 teaspoon goji berries, soaked for 10 minutes
- 1 teaspoon chia seeds
- 1 cup unsweetened organic coconut milk
- water to adjust consistency to personal preference

DIRECTIONS

1. Combine all ingredients in a blender and puree until smooth and thick.
2. Enjoy!

Hemp Green Smoothie

INGREDIENTS

- 2 ounces of spinach
- 2 ounces of kale
- 1 ounce of hemp seeds
- 1 large of banana
- 1.5-2 cups of water

DIRECTIONS

1. Combine all ingredients in a blender and puree until smooth and thick.
2. Enjoy!

Avocado Green Smoothie

INGREDIENTS

- 8 ounce unsweetened almond milk
- 2-3 cups spinach
- 1 medium banana, peeled
- 1/2 small avocado

DIRECTIONS

1. Combine all ingredients in a blender and puree until smooth and thick.
2. Enjoy!

Super Green Smoothie

INGREDIENTS

- 2 cups Kale
- 1 cucumber
- 1 stalk of celery
- 2 cups frozen fruit chunks (peaches, mango, pineapple)
- 1 frozen banana, peeled
- 1/2 small avocado
- 1 lemon, peeled
- 16 ounces water

DIRECTIONS

1. Combine all ingredients in a blender and puree until smooth and thick.
2. Enjoy!

Pineapple-Strawberry Green Smoothie

INGREDIENTS

- 1 and 1/2 cups kale
- 1/2 cup parsley
- 2 cups fresh pineapple
- 1 cups whole strawberries
- 1 medium banana, peeled
- 1 Tablespoon Hemp seeds

DIRECTIONS

1. Combine all ingredients in a blender and puree until smooth and thick.
2. Enjoy!

Fruit and Almond Smoothie

INGREDIENTS

- 1 cup original Almond milk
- 1 cup frozen strawberries and peaches
- 1-3.5 ounce Greek Yogurt

DIRECTIONS

1. Combine all ingredients in a blender and puree until smooth and thick.
2. Enjoy!

Ice Cold Banana and Mango Smoothie

INGREDIENTS

- 1/2 banana
- 1/2 peeled and chopped mango
- 1/2 cup Greek yogurt
- 2/3 cup skimmed milk
- Some ice cubes
- 2 teaspoon of protein powder

DIRECTIONS

1. Combine all ingredients in a blender and puree until smooth and thick.
2. Enjoy!

Lime and Spinach Smoothie

INGREDIENTS

- Juice of 4 limes
- Zest of 2 of the limes
- 2 cups spinach leaves
- 1 tablespoon of sunflower butter
- Several ice cubes

DIRECTIONS

1. Combine all ingredients in a blender and puree until smooth and thick.
2. Enjoy!

Blueberry-Almond Smoothie

INGREDIENTS

- 1-½ cup blueberries
- 1 cup ice cubes
- 1/2 cup plain Greek yogurt
- ¼ cup slivered almonds
- 2 tablespoon wheat germ
- 2 tablespoon skim milk or unsweetened almond milk
- 2 tablespoon honey

DIRECTIONS

1. Combine all ingredients in a blender and puree until smooth and thick.
2. Enjoy!

Pina Colada Smoothie

INGREDIENTS

- 1 cup light plain yogurt
- 1 cup fresh or canned pineapple (cut into small chunks)
- 1 teaspoon coconut extract
- 1 cup crushed ice

DIRECTIONS

1. Combine all ingredients in a blender and puree until smooth and thick.
2. Enjoy!

Low-Carb Green Tea Smoothie

INGREDIENTS

- 2 teaspoon Matcha green tea powder
- 3 tablespoons hot water
- 1 banana (cut into small chunks)
- 1 package sugar substitute
- 1 cup skim milk
- 1 cup crushed ice
- 1 teaspoon mint extract (optional)

DIRECTIONS

1. Mix green tea powder with hot water and stir until it forms a paste. Add the green tea paste and the other ingredients to a blender and process until smooth.
2. Serve and enjoy!

Mean Green Diabetic Smoothie

INGREDIENTS

- 2 cups fresh spinach
- 1/2 apple, sliced
- 1/2 avocado
- 1 cup unsweetened almond milk
- 3 tablespoon Greek yogurt
- 1 tablespoon flax seeds
- 1 teaspoon vanilla extract
- 1/2 cup ice cubes

DIRECTIONS

1. In a powerful blender, combine ingredients and blend until smooth. Add more almond milk if necessary to reach desired consistency.
2. Serve immediately.

Blueberry Flax Yogurt Smoothie

INGREDIENTS

- ¾ cup fresh or frozen blueberries
- ½ eight inch banana, chilled
- 1 (6 ounces) Greek yogurt
- 1 tablespoon ground flax seeds

DIRECTIONS

1. Combine all ingredients in a blender and puree until smooth and thick.
2. Enjoy!

Peach Smoothie

INGREDIENTS

- 2 cups soymilk
- 2 medium bananas
- 4 medium peaches
- 1/2 teaspoon ground cinnamon

DIRECTIONS

1. Combine all ingredients in a blender and puree until smooth and thick.
2. Enjoy!

Berry Blast Smoothie

INGREDIENTS

- 1 cup almond milk
- 1 frozen banana
- 1 1/2 cups of berries
- 1 cup of water

DIRECTIONS

1. Combine all ingredients in a blender and puree
   until smooth and thick.
2. Enjoy!

Banana & Mango Smoothie

INGREDIENTS

- 1/2 banana
- 1/2 peeled and chopped mango
- 1/2 cup Greek yogurt
- 2/3 cup almond milk

DIRECTIONS

1. Combine all ingredients in a blender and puree until smooth and thick.
2. Enjoy!

Strawberry-Banana-Flax Smoothie

INGREDIENTS

- 1-1/2 cups fresh strawberries, trimmed
- 1/2 medium banana, sliced
- 2 tablespoons ground flax seeds
- 2 tablespoons almond milk (unsweetened)
- 2 teaspoons honey
- 1 cup ice cubes

DIRECTIONS

1. Combine all ingredients in a blender and puree until smooth and thick.
2. Enjoy!

Mango Blueberry Smoothie

INGREDIENTS

- 1 mango
- A handful of frozen blueberries
- 1 bunch of dandelion greens
- 1/4 teaspoon ground cinnamon
- 2 cups of pure or filtered water

DIRECTIONS

1. Combine all ingredients in a blender and puree until smooth and thick.
2. Enjoy!

Fresh Parsley, Goji, and Grapefruit Smoothie

INGREDIENTS

- 2 tablespoons goji berries
- 1/2 grapefruit, peeled and seeded
- 2 tablespoons ground flaxseed
- 1 tablespoon coconut oil
- 1-1/2 cups water
- 1 cup parsley, loosely packed
- 1/2 cup baby spinach, loosely packed

DIRECTIONS

1. Place the goji berries in a bowl with 1/4 cup of room temperature water. Place in the fridge to soak for at least 20 minutes or overnight.
2. Combine the goji berries, grapefruit, flaxseed, coconut oil, and water in the blender and secure the lid.
3. Starting at low speed and gradually increasing toward high, blend the ingredients for 1 minute or until the mixture contains no visible pieces of fruit.
4. Add the parsley and spinach and blend again at medium speed for 30 seconds, gradually increasing the speed to high. Blend on high speed for another 15 to 30 seconds or until the entire mixture is smooth.
5. Pour the smoothie into two glasses and enjoy!

Conclusion

Thank you for reading. If you want to read my other books you can go to Amazon and check my author page.

If you've enjoyed this book, I would like you to leave a positive review on Amazon. If you want to add something and have some suggestions write them down.

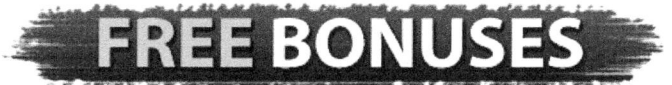

FREE BONUSES

Every copy of this book comes packed with 2 invaluable bonuses for diabetics and pre-diabetics:

BONUS #1: *Step-By-Step Blueprint **"6 Steps To Reverse Diabetes Naturally And Have A Perfect Health"** - FREE INSTANT DOWNLOAD*
BONUS #2: *Our exclusive newsletter subscription where we share tips, strategies and support to destroy diabetes once and for all - FREE INSTANT ACCESS*

Simply visit the special link below and enter your name & email address to get instant access.

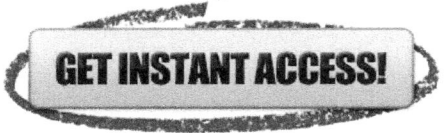

WWW.SOURCEOFHEALTHY.COM/6STEPS

Thank you! Keep living healthy!

Made in the USA
Monee, IL
05 March 2021